Everything Will Be Alright

Everything Will Be Alright

✦

An Alzheimer's Memoir

by glory read

iUniverse, Inc.

New York Lincoln Shanghai

Everything Will Be Alright
An Alzheimer's Memoir

iUniverse books may be ordered through booksellers or by contacting:

iUniverse
2021 Pine Lake Road, Suite 100
Lincoln, NE 68512
www.iuniverse.com
1-800-Authors (1-800-288-4677)

Front cover picture—Spring break at Myrtle Beach, South Carolina
Cover Design by William M. Read, IV

ISBN: 978-0-595-44006-1 (pbk)
ISBN: 978-0-595-68762-6 (cloth)
ISBN: 978-0-595-88327-1 (ebk)

Printed in the United States of America

To Bill

who loved me and believed that I could do anything

and to the family we made

Contents

Introduction

There are many stories that attest to the power of love and commitment to triumph over the dark times of life.

To understand this phenomenon requires an intimate knowledge of the players, and that is how this book evolved.

It is a personal account of how my husband and I were able to transcend the challenges of Alzheimer's disease and grow closer to each other during our shared eleven-year experience.

It is our love story.

Bill's emotions far outlived his memory even after awareness seemed to be gone. Our perception of the disease and the power of love, commitment and emotional courage changed the dynamics of the disease for us.

Everyone's experience is different, but we can all call on the human spirit for help. Utilizing our inner resources to fight Alzheimer's made it possible for us to weather this sad disease with dignity and love.

It is my hope that our experience may provide insight and inspiration for others.

Prologue

Our tree is gone.

The Cherry Blossom tree my husband Bill planted for me thirty-something years ago is no longer proudly standing in front of our home.

When I looked out the window one summer morning, it had mysteriously disappeared. I was in shock.

It was a survivor, even after it had been hit by a speeding car with a driver under the influence some years ago. Its injury was only that it leaned to the right, and it bravely continued to greet spring with its glorious blossoms.

Our sentimental tree had met its untimely death at the hands of men wearing orange vests. No one asked me, called me, or gave an explanation of "why". Our tree was not dead. It may have been ill and may have needed pruning, but now all that is left is a stump and shavings. It was assassinated.

My sons mourn with me.

Our tree is gone.

PART I
The End

My ability to visualize that day is blurred by the preceding three or four days when my husband Bill would breath and then stop breathing while those of us at his bedside counted the intervals and prayed that his suffering would soon end. Through intermittent tears and numbness, I became aware that his handsome face needed shaving and his fingernails needed clipping because I had put off these things not wanting to add to his discomfort.

Memories of his death come back to me in bits and pieces without continuity. It was early morning and the sun was beaming after many days of dark dreary skies, and I sat on our bed that was beside the hospital bed where I had been sleeping—or trying to sleep—since his final decline had begun five months earlier.

He was where he wanted to be, in our home in Clifton, New Jersey with me and the family we had made. Our sons, Bill and Phil, our teenage grandchildren, Lauren, Philip Jr., Leanna, and Keirsten, and their moms, Nancy and Donna were there for us.

It was almost the kind of end that had become one of my goals for him during the eleven years that we lived with the saddest disease—Alzheimer's.

But we were blessed that despite Bill's clouded mind and the morphine of his last days, he was able to recognize me and our immediate family and to manage his famous smile.

At other times, as he wandered in and out of his delusionary state, he had asked, "Will you marry me?", and when I told him we had been married for 49 years, he would smile, saying, "You're my best girl, green eyes."

As he was dying I became aware of his treasured Duke class ring which had become a permanent identification. Our alma mater is where we began our life journey together, but the Alzheimer's years brought us closer to each other. His spirit made it possible for him to say "I love you" until the inevitable end. All along the way there were rainbows of enlightenment that gave me a greater appreciation of what marriage and family are really all about.

When his disease was obviously entering the final stage but he was still able to interact with us as much as his clouded mind could manage, he suddenly developed a high fever. At the hospital emergency room, he was diagnosed with an infected gall bladder that had to be removed. He came through the operation, but the anesthetic probably advanced his Alzheimer's. After several weeks in the hospital, he returned home bedridden.

The dying process was beginning, and our world inside became as dark as the weather outside. Cold winter rain beat against the window panes and the swaying pine tree tossed snow morsels against them.

My heart ached as the process moved through Bill's November birthday, Thanksgiving, our son Bill's December birthday and our wedding anniversary in March.

Throughout this time, I sat by his bed holding his trembling hands and soothing his brow and our pain was shared. I held his hand tightly so I could physically feel our connection.

He would squeeze my hand in response.

When my tears were ready to flow I would go downstairs, have a glass of wine, stare at the television, walk around aimlessly—and then return to his side.

That year, a small version of our annual Christmas Eve buffet was only for our small family. There was no Christmas tree for the first time, but Phil put up a string of tiny white lights on the evergreen tree that stands in front of the living room picture window.

Being together helped all of us cope. But I felt guilty that he couldn't be down stairs to share this time with us.

Bill's ever-ready smile of appreciation when our granddaughters kissed him or Phil came by after his morning run or he greeted Bill with, "hello my son" were the rainbows that gave meaning to the last days of his life and helped sustain us through the darkest days.

The time leading up to his death was raw pain that never ceased as I walked through the fog of his deterioration. His difficulty swallowing limited his already reduced diet of Jell-O, milk shakes, and chocolate pudding to dwindle to ice cream. I gave him water with an eyedropper.

We had a live-in aide from the time he returned home from the hospital because I was unable to move him. His legs were rigid and every movement caused him terrible pain, but even so he would always thank her for helping him.

The last month of his life he was on hospice program that provided the morphine to dull his pain so he was able to sleep for brief periods until his last days when he sometimes slipped into semi consciousness with his eyes open. He fought death—everyone's right—throughout the five months that he remained bed-ridden.

Toward the end, my emotions had become so jumbled; I didn't want him to suffer any more, but I couldn't bear for him to die. Bill gave me unconditional love, he nursed my self-esteem and he was my fan club. He was my anchor and our home was our haven. How could I live without my best friend? All the limitation and endless problems didn't seem to matter anymore, but it was too late.

William Marsden Read III died on April 2, 2001.

His death was so unreal to me that I found myself playing the role of hostess at the funeral home visitation. His friends were coming to visit him, but he wasn't there. If there had not been a crowd I would have been angry, but I didn't have to worry because the crowds came and I rose to the occasion by making sure I spoke with everyone. I directed them to the photo display and told them the story associated with each picture.

Because Bill never talked about himself and his accomplishments, I had always been his "press agent." Now I fell into the public relations role I was playing. Later when I asked myself "what was I thinking?" I realized that I was on automatic and my emotions were not surfacing.

When I touched his ice-cold hand in the funeral home, a chill ran right through my bones. It wasn't Bill. I found it hard to even look at him again, but I needed to confirm that it was him.

At the church service my mind was not aware of what was actually happening. It was as if I was in a strange place at an event that I didn't recognize—but my sons, Bill and Phil were up there talking about their father. They talked about when he was their Cub Scout master and about the love he earned from his neighbors. The few words that got through to me were Bill saying, "he always saw the good in people," and "he gave us the gift of his smile." Phil said, "he had a wonderful life," and thanked him for "making our life wonderful too." I thought they had captured the essence of him, but they looked so sad.

Reality briefly hit me as we followed the casket out of the church and we got into the limo, and saw so many friends standing around.

I don't remember the short ride after the service to the cemetery in Upper Montclair, N.J. even though we drove by our home for the last time together. At the cemetery, I only have a vague recollection of being handed a rose and the folded flag. It was almost a total blur.

My numbness was protecting me from reality.

My only real memory was a flashback to the time when we bought the cemetery plot one summer day about five years earlier. It was a glorious day and we joked about always wanting to own property in Upper Montclair. We chose a plot in Mt. Hebron Cemetery close to Valley Road where Montclair University students parked their cars and a nearby church with a nursery school playground where little children at play could be heard.

Baby squirrels scampered across the paths as they enjoyed their own playground. It was an alive place with sunlight dancing through the branches of the big trees. To add to the perfect cemetery, the writer of one of our favorite songs, "As Time Goes By" was buried there.

Bill did not seem to recognize the purchase as imminent, and I pushed the thought away.

Then we went and had a strawberry ice cream cone at Applegate Farm.

My early visits to his grave gave me some comfort until I began visualizing his body decaying in the ground. Some times I felt a "crazy" urge to get down on my knees and dig him up with my hands.

There was an untapped reservoir of tears inside of me. Usually, I only cry on the inside, but later these tears would erupt at unexpected times and for unrelated reasons.

I stopped going to the cemetery for a brief time. When I began going again, I took plants in our favorite colors, red for him and lilac for me. From our yard I took huge white blossoms with an intoxicating aroma that were from a southern magnolia bush Bill had brought back on the plane after a summer at Duke for a special computer programming course. It took many years for the magnolia to adapt to a northern climate and become a tree that is higher than our house—and spreads its essence in the neighborhood. At Christmas, I always put a mini ever-green tree on his grave.

At the cemetery, waves of sadness and despair washed over me as I sat up toppled flowers on nearby graves because it was what Bill would have done. Some days I tarried to enjoy the view of the Manhattan sky-line trying to vicariously share the pleasures he was missing.

PART II
Bill and Glory

The southern late-fall sun warmed me as I left my pre-lunch Journalism class and walked across the quad in front of the chapel to meet a girl friend at the cafeteria on the men's campus of Duke University. This campus and the women's campus are a couple of miles apart with a stretch of natural beauty and some faculty homes connecting them.

My friend needed a lunch companion to keep her real mission from being too obvious. She was on a quest to meet every guy on campus, and I abetted her by letting her buy my lunch. She wasn't the only coed who planned her classes on the basis of meeting guys by selecting courses that were only taught on the men's campus.

At that time in history, the '40s, most of the female students were there because their elite families wanted to prepare them to be "suitable wives" for the future doctors and lawyers they would meet at Duke's top medical and law schools, and would later marry.

We all looked alike in our skirts and sweaters and loafers, but I didn't fit in this category by pedigree.

My family background was different and not conventional compared to most coeds, but I appreciated college's promise for my future. It empowered me with the promise that I could make my life the way I imagined it could be.

My mind was not on marriage.

My quasi-friend was a freshman, pretty and rich, and I was a sophomore. She was bright enough to be accepted to prestigious Duke but her obvious interest was not academic, and she only survived that one year. She probably had no time to study. I have often wondered what happened to her. Did she become a corporate wife, did she have a string of failed marriages, or did she become an author of romance novels? I hope she had a good life.

When I passed other students basking in the sun as they lounged on the chapel steps, I spotted my friend already in the lunch line that spilled out of the dining room building chatting with a couple of cute guys.

When she introduced me to Bill, I couldn't help but notice his incredible smile, open and honest like a child's. There was warmth in his voice but it was only when I looked into his warm gray-blue eyes that seemed to look right into my soul that I wanted to know him better. My feeling of connection was more than I was willing to admit to myself that day.

I didn't know that I had just met my future.

My views on dating at that time were probably similar to most of the guys who were serious students but wanted to have a social life too.

The ones who were not still in uniform were returning from service in World War II. They were from all over the country, and those of northern origin perceived some of us as "sweet southern girls," which enhanced our popularity; I was enjoying being in the midst of a wonderful social life when I met Bill.

My freshman year had ended on VE (victory Europe) Day, which happened to be my birthday. Everyone believed that there would never be another world war as we rode down the streets in open convertibles with horns blaring to celebrate.

Bill was a product of the officer training program, and when I met him he had just returned to Duke after serving in the Pacific Theater as a Lieutenant on a troop landing ship.

At seventeen, he had begun college as a civilian, joined the deferred draft Navy V12 program and graduated from officer training school at Northwestern University before actively serving in the war.

The two-year deferred draft program saved young men who were already in college from being drafted at eighteen and sent directly to war. They were in uniform and actually in the service, taking a combination of academic and military courses and under a military ten o'clock curfew. Any infractions of academic or behavior rules meant that the deal was off and they were immediately shipped off to active duty.

When the veterans returned to campus, college life was not the same and they were more mature and serious students as they tried to pick up their lives. Many of them had educational funds from the GI bill, a benefit for World War II veterans.

Bill returned to Duke remembered as the chemistry major who had made the highest chemistry placement score in the university's history when he was a pre-war freshman. He was eager to continue his science courses and to begin a graduate program in his academic pursuits when we met.

Ironically, I had just realized that I had better give up physical sciences after a troublesome episode when I accidentally created a misting odor that made it necessary for the class to evacuate the lab. Everyone was coughing and looking around trying to find the culprit. To add to my embarrassment, Bill later told me "Your lab instructor is my friend who is working with me on a research project."

Bill asked me, "What happened in the chem. lab?"

"I don't know," I truthfully replied, "I just don't get chemistry."

"It's easy, I'll help you," he promised.

And, he tried, but it didn't seem to help. Maybe I was subconsciously being nagged by my desire to write. So I decided to turn to the only Journalism class offered. The great professor had been a foreign correspondent and was now on his retirement career. The small class produced several successful writers. I was the only girl in the class and the dating prospects looked good, but I met Bill before they materialized.

When Bill called me the night after our meeting to invite me to the upcoming big campus dance, I was excited about the quick attention. On our first date at a popular campus hangout a couple of days later, I tripped and fell as he was helping me across the street. I blamed him, but I wasn't going to give up the invitation to the big dance. He was handsome, and even this early I couldn't deny the romantic attachment I already felt for him.

On that first date our conversation was casual as we talked about our classes, and he teased me, "Your eyes match my car," he said, referring to the old green Roadmaster Buick that was on loan to him from his family.

Our frequent dates soon turned into spending all of our free time together. When we weren't studying or taking advantage of all the social opportunities of campus life, we talked about everything, from our philosophy of life to campus gossip.

Dancing to the live big bands like Glen Miller, playing those romantic songs of our era was the beginning of our love of dancing together that helped move our romance along. It was magical to glide across the dance floor in my favorite black strapless gown with the tiny sequins that sparkled like stars, and Bill so handsome in his tuxedo. It was like being alone in a surreal place with his smile embracing me.

For me, there had never been anyone that I had been able to open up to. The intensity when he looked into my eyes, reminiscent of our first meeting, made me quickly learn to trust him and to believe that he would never betray me. My feeling of happiness was encompassing, but I analyzed my feelings because I was about to give away my heart.

When Bill gave me his fraternity pin a couple of months after we met, we became a couple. As was the custom, his frat brothers serenaded me, and Bill told me, "I knew it had to be you the day I met you," paraphrasing the popular song.

As our affinity grew, we became a serious college romance meeting between classes every day and sitting on the base of the founder's statue for endless conversations about everything.

Discovering what a special person Bill was reinforced my feelings of being loved and secure, filling a void of my earlier life.

Our campus gossip began when Bill told me that he had been invited with a few other students to the home of his mentor chemistry professor.

When I inquired about how the visit went Bill said, "You'll never guess what it was like. It was enlightening as I expected—even with the distraction of laundry hanging in the living room which was in view of the meeting in the den." We laughed as we tried to understand this peculiarity. When Bill asked, "Tell me your best story," I told the story about my political science professor. He definitely had it in for me because he considered my first name to be a nickname and, to add to that black mark, was his observation of Bill and I kissing just before his class. Information he revealed to the class.

This professor was not a romantic and he was volatile, throwing books across the room when he got annoyed, and flunking students for illegitimate reasons. I passed in spite of my handicaps and I consider that course enlightening about politics—and people.

But my most interesting story was about my charismatic psychology professor who shocked everyone by seeming to prove the prevailing idea that all psychology professors are "crazy", even though he had not previously fit the description. He was movie-star handsome, married to a beautiful woman, and had a couple of adorable children. He was a super teacher and kind and parental to his students. We all loved him.

Out of the blue came the revelation when we began seeing him ride around in an open red convertible with an older woman (deemed unattractive). He soon disappeared and the last news we got was that he was divorced. We never knew the "why" or the end of the story. It was Psychology 101 in action and the talk of the campus.

Bill and I spent all our time together, studying in the library, and often having dinner on "spaghetti night" at a boarding house just off campus that was frequented by medical and graduate students. "Mom Cross" and her family ran the place and were famous for allowing students to run up a tab when they were short on cash. Or we would "dine" in a little place near the campus where the genial proprietor allowed us to sit for hours with a hamburger and a beer. We talked volumes there, and it became "our place."

I had never invited friends to dinner with my family because I was reluctant to have them see our humble lifestyle, but I finally decided that I had to invite Bill. My Mom was already suffering from cancer, but she made her wonderful pot roast.

Bill was completely at ease, and it was an important step for our future life together by brining him into my family. He grew to love my Mom, and later tried to understand my father.

Our first separation was when Bill went home to New Jersey for semester break. On the phone he urged me to join him at his parents' for the rest of the school break, but it was one of his daily letters that gave me impetus to accept the invitation. The letter read, "I didn't get home until 4 AM from Daily's Meadowbrook (a famous spot in Cedar Grove, N.J. that featured big bands and was especially popular with college students). I was there with a family friend, but I was good, and only thinking of you."

The blizzard of 1947 began as I boarded a train to New Jersey to meet Bill's family. It seemed like such a long time since we had seen each other that nothing was going to stop me from taking that trip.

When I arrived at Penn Station in New York the historic blizzard was in full force, and I waited there watching the swirling snow beat against the waiting room windows for the two hours it took Bill to travel twelve short miles from Maywood, N.J. to pick me up and two more hours before we got back to his family's home.

We got stuck in the snow twice but were in a high mood as we kissed with the snow whirling around us because it was so good to see each other again. Bill wrapped his arms around me to shield me from the cold and said, "we'll never be apart again."

It was a promise that he always tried to keep.

I had never seen so much snow, but I was anxious to meet his family that I thought would be a family to me someday.

We spent the rest of the time sleigh riding in the little park where he showed me his name on a bronze plaque honoring local men who had served in World War II.

We returned to Duke together on the train.

Our backgrounds were so very different.

Bill grew up in Maywood, N.J., a pretty little village but unlike the posh ones that are prevalent in the state; it is a middle-class community in northern New Jersey with easy access to New York City.

His father commuted to his job as an accountant at Chase Manhattan Bank headquarters on Wall Street in the city, and his mother stayed home with the children.

Bill was the oldest, and weighed less than three pounds when he was born but grew to health in an improvised incubator and was fed with the inside of a fountain pen. He always felt gratitude for his good health.

His was a typical suburban childhood. He was interested in art and photography as well as science, and had a dark room and a chemistry lab in the basement. As the oldest of the three children, Bill met his parents' expectations of babysitting his siblings, and helping his father with chores and home repairs.

In high school he won four recognitions in the yearbook, most artistic, friendliest, popular and best disposition. He enjoyed the cultural and social life of teens who live so close to the Big Apple.

During summers, he worked in labs at nearby chemical companies, and his high school chemistry teacher became his mentor and was instrumental in Bill's acceptance to Duke when he was seventeen.

I was born in the row house of my mother's friend in Baltimore, Maryland. My parents were passing through on the way south. At the time, my father was a part owner of a carnival and they were on their way to winter headquarters.

My colorful childhood was spent with children of acrobats, clowns, concessionaires, aerialists and exotic dancers. Our days were filled with free rides, junk food, and sneaking under a tent to see someone's mother dance like Salome. In Florida where we wintered with circus people I learned how to walk the tight rope.

We were nomadic, moving every week from fair to fair in all the towns and hamlets in New York, Pennsylvania, New Jersey—the entire northeast region. I only have a vague memory of any of these places but I remember always getting carsick.

My father's "career" had its ups and downs so we moved back and forth from being really poor to almost rich. My early childhood passed with my erred perception of my life as "normal."

I finally started school at the age of eight, when my mother convinced my father that not only did I need a formal education but that they could be arrested if I didn't go to school. Each year I attended at least two different schools in different parts of the country. It was a fragmented education for a lonely child with no siblings, scant relatives, no roots, and no real home.

These years awakened me to the reality that my life was different than that of other children, and the knowledge introduced me to the feeling of being an "alien."

My knowledge of my first generation Irish father, Michael Joseph Meehan, is sketchy.

I learned that before his carnival years, he had been a minor league baseball player and a vaudeville entertainer. He was born in Troy, New York, but left home in his teens and lied to enlist in the Army to fight uprisings in the Philippine Islands. With no formal education, he read the encyclopedia and the dictionary, an activity he shared with me. He utilized his native intelligence and gift of gab to earn a living.

Some additional light was shed on my father's mysterious history when he located his three siblings who had not heard from him in many years in the Bronx in New York. I don't know how he found them. His brother was a guide at the Metropolitan Museum of Art, one sister was a private nurse to a wealthy widow who lived in The Plaza Hotel and gave us glassware with the Plaza logo on them, and the other sister was the family home keeper. They lived together in a large apartment building with a pretty flowering courtyard right in front of their windows. There is a lone picture of me standing in the courtyard holding my doll when I was about six years old.

They had no children and I was embraced by them. I reveled in the attention, as did my mother.

They took us to see the sights in Manhattan, to the top of the Empire State Building, and to a Radio City Music Hall show.

At Christmases they sent us a big package filled with "goodies" to eat, toys, and fashionable clothes for my model-slim mother, all from the famous Wanamaker Department Store when the Bronx was a fashionable borough. The packages came to a P.O. Box wherever we happened to be at the time.

For several years, we visited them about once a year and I don't know when or why the relationship disappeared, but I missed the family feeling, and New York.

Many years later I tried to locate them, without success. I had hoped that I might find some clues to my genealogy.

I know even less about my quiet gentle mother, Margaret Hill, whose parents died when she was still a young child, and she spent her life shuffled from stepparent to stepparent, living in Florida or North Carolina.

After my father married the eighteen year old, southern girl, who was fifteen years younger than he was, and I was born, our nomadic family life began. It continued until my mother was diagnosed with tuberculosis. She was in her thirties and I was thirteen years old.

Her departure for isolation in the sanitarium in Black Mountain, N.C. where she would spend the next four years, was a surprise to me because no one told me of her illness to prepare me. It was so abrupt that she just seemed to disappear—and my world caved in.

For me, it was as if she had died.

My father was traveling, and I felt abandoned by him.

My aunt Jo saved me from an orphanage when I went to live with her in Durham, N.C., where we had visited occasionally.

I was not allowed to visit my mother during these years when she was in the sanitarium because of the virulence of the disease in those days.

My memories of these events are vague because I blocked them out, but the trauma changed my life dramatically—and left scars on my psyche.

After she returned from the sanitarium my mother, the stranger, and I talked about her stay there to try to catch up on those years that we were separated.

She told me about a doctor, who was also a patient, who had turned her into an avid reader, beginning with the books of Thomas Wolfe, who had lived in the area.

Reading hadn't become my life companion until the summer of my thirteenth year when my mother first went away. I spent that entire summer, all my waking hours, curled up in an old big soft chair in the hallway of my aunt's house engrossed in books of all kinds. I rarely spoke to anyone.

It was the ultimate escape from my life when I was in such bad shape emotionally. I got lost in all kinds of books that I borrowed from the library. There were so many books, so long ago, that I would have to research my mind to compile any kind of list of favorites. It was the time in my life that I fell in love with words, and I still don't think that there is any form of communication as antidotal as the printed word.

Television was in its infancy when my Mom came home and she visited her sister to watch television, as was a custom of many people. Visiting someone fortunate enough to have a set was a social event like visiting someone to play bridge.

Another patient, a priest, became my mother's friend and converted her to Roman Catholicism and when she returned home she wanted to be married in the church. My parents had been married in a civil ceremony and my father was okay with her desire although he was not a churchgoer—so the three of us went to the local parish for the ceremony. It was important to my mother who practiced her faith for the rest of her life.

When I try to understand my parents' lives I usually come to the conclusion that they were victims of their circumstances. I can't judge them because I barely got to know them.

Even though I don't have warm fuzzy memories of my childhood, I do believe that they loved me. During their illnesses, I was able to make the kind of peace with them that I needed.

My high school years were about raising myself. Emotionally "needy," I was drawn to activities that gained recognition and made me feel appreciated. I found it in starring in dramas, like "The Necklace," which got me rave reviews in the local daily newspaper. They also printed my poems about war because of their timeliness.

As high school female students during war time, we all went to USO (united service organization) dances at the local club frequented by ROTC and Navy V12 Duke students and the Army basic trainees from nearby Ft. Bragg.

In this period of theatrical ambitions, I also became a member of the chorus line of a show put together by a student with show biz aspirations that entertained at the Army camp. The soldiers appreciated our cancan, especially when the costumes began to unravel, and I even got to "talk" a sultry song when the usual singer was a no-show.

After high school I was beginning to adjust to living with my parents again, and without concrete plans for my future. I continued patriotic (everyone was patriotic then) activities by serving almost-fulltime as a volunteer Red Cross nurse's aide in the hospital, and donating my O negative blood—whenever I was able to meet the hundred pound weight requirement.

After a series of the terrible jobs available for high school graduates who couldn't type, I found a no-brainer job at Duke Hospital that was the beginning of important life changes. My personal life was in limbo but my motivation was growing, and I had developed inner self-confidence, and I was resilient.

The year of working at Duke Hospital between high school and college was a time of getting myself together and increasing my self confidence.

Keeping records in the lab didn't require much brainpower, but it offered other rewards. I liked wearing a lab coat and unofficially watching operations, and I began reading textbooks available in the lab.

But the real benefit was the lab technicians and medical students, who were only a few years older than me, but adopted me as a "sister." They taught me how to do lab tests and they took me along to their local hangout where they drank beer and talked shop—and I became fascinated with their world. They encouraged and convinced me that I had to enroll in college.

It took my honest essay revealing my unconventional earlier life, and my determined aspirations for my future, which were not yet specific but strong, to get me accepted to Duke.

It was when I was in the registration line that I realized how ill prepared I was compared to the other freshmen who had been academically at the top in their high schools.

The big question was how to pay the tuition. There were no such things as student loans, my academic record didn't qualify me for any of the few scholarships available, and my family was poor. But, I somehow managed with savings from the year I had worked, part-time jobs, and jobs I had during school breaks and summers.

PART III
Our Life Together

Storm clouds that would delay our future were already beginning to gather over my family situation while Bill and I were still in college. It was the onset of a period of time that distracted us from our studies and the fun period of our romance. As we continued to pursue our goals our life became more serious and apprehensive, and our conversations were about my family's situation.

My mother had only been home a couple of years from the sanitarium where she had been during my early adolescence, and my father had to stop traveling because of his ill health.

When my father's illness was diagnosed as bone marrow cancer, Bill's whole fraternity donated blood.

My mother had become my father's caretaker, and I spent more time with them—and Bill got to know them better.

Then my mother was diagnosed with cancer, which was temporarily arrested by an operation. They were in and out of the hospital, sometimes there at the same time. The trips were to stabilize them. My mother was treated with radiation, and my father with blood transfusions. There was no chemotherapy at that time.

It was becoming such a chaotic time that I wondered why Bill didn't just run. But he didn't, as he assured me "I'll always be here to help you."

He was there for me and provided the emotional support that saved me from despair during the following two-year period when my father died and my mother had a reoccurrence of her cancer that would defeat her while she was still in her forties.

My care giving and financial help were needed more than ever. While my friends were working on their career paths, I was trying to deal with life's big issues—death, illness and finances.

By this time Bill was taking a few graduate courses and working part time as an engineering draftsman at city hall and for an architect, postponing some of his ambitions to be able to help me.

I was working at the newspaper writing feature articles, which I loved, but at the same time trying to deal with my mother's worsened condition. Her sister, my Aunt Jo, and volunteers from my Mom's church were caring for her in shifts. Bill or I would often spend the night on a cot in her tiny apartment so she would not be alone.

We kept postponing marriage in the hope that things would somehow improve—but they only got worse.

Finally, we just decided to stop waiting for better days—and got married.

There was no white wedding dress, no lavish party and no glamorous honeymoon.

But it was a beautiful warm first day of spring, March 20, when the chaplain to the students at the University of North Carolina, two observing divinity students, and two of our friends gathered in the tiny ancient church, Chapel of the Cross, in Chapel Hill, North Carolina, where we made our wedding vows. I wore a blue suit and corsage Bill gave me—and he said, "You're beautiful."

We didn't need the trappings to know that our commitment was forever, symbolized by the plain gold circle of the rings we exchanged. Bill had been the keeper of these rings for such a long time that they had imprinted circles on the leather of his wallet.

He had not been able to afford an engagement ring when we first talked of marriage so he had the fraternity pin with tiny pearls and rubies made into a still-treasured ring that I wore on my third finger left hand. During later more affluent years Bill always "nagged" me to pick out a diamond but it was of no importance to me, I loved the statement of the lone gold circle that has never left my finger. Bill's is still with him.

With trials still ahead of us, we moved into our three-room apartment in a large complex where many married Duke students lived. There were four apartments in each of some twenty buildings, and ours was across the street from Durham's most famous barbecue restaurant that permeated the air with tempting odors, and when we felt that we could "splurge" Bill would pick up a takeout order for us.

There had been so many delays that we felt as if we were behind in our life plans. And we were eager to start a family, which was such an important part of our commitment. We called upon our courage because we didn't want to put anything on hold again.

My mother was in the dying process during my first pregnancy. She had just returned home from one of her hospital stays when I went into the hospital for my first Cesarean section.

At that time in history C-sections were treated like any other major surgery. I was completely anesthetized and remained in the hospital for ten days even though there were no complications for me, or our baby.

I didn't get to see our first son, William M. Read, IV for many hours, but it didn't dampen the joy of this great privilege life had given us. Bill's happiness was evident to the entire maternity floor of Duke Hospital as he waited outside the operating room to greet our son. The ultimate life experience is to grow a human being inside your own body, and for us, no other event would ever compare to the intensity and indescribable feeling of having made a person. The life-long commitment it entails cements the parental bond in a unique way and forever.

When I returned from the recovery room, Bill was waiting with roses and his incredible smile. Our best dream was a reality; we were making a family.

On our way home from the hospital we stopped by her apartment for my bedridden mother to see her first grandson for the only time. As ill as she was, there was joy on her face—she had lived for this.

On our first Christmas Eve as a family Bill was with my mother (so her sister could be with her family) and I was in our little haven walking our colicky son. How could there be a better husband?

A few weeks later my mother died.

Bill and I were visiting her in the hospital and didn't know it would be the last time we would see her alive. Without any signs of distress, she said "I'm going to die", and quickly died.

I have no understanding of this scene or what my immediate reaction was—except "unreal." As we were leaving the hospital, I vaguely remember bumping into a medical student we knew, who asked, "How are you?" I said, "My mother just died."

When my father had died earlier, I was at the nursing home with my mother. My father looked like a skeleton and was coherent but unaware of his condition. My poor mother looked so bad that I went to get coffee for her, and when I returned she told me he had died.

I have no recollection of either of their funerals.

I have wondered if my parents' illnesses and deaths had set my reaction to my husband's death—not a reality.

Bill told me, "You and your Mom were stoic," an accusation he recanted when he learned how to read my emotions when there were no tears to help wash away the pain.

My Mom and I both internalized our pain to have a brave front for emotional survival. It was more painful than shedding tears, and I often longed for my tears to flow.

Mourning for my mother was more about the life she didn't get to live instead of the short one she spent fighting her diseases. Sadly, I didn't get enough time to really know my Mom.

After my mother's death, Bill and I and our baby son began the process of restructuring.

We struggled to reach more financial stability and to begin a more peaceful life as a family. Bill got a full time job as a chemist at the local water department, and I had time to appreciate the joys of motherhood, as I did free-lance feature writing for North Carolina newspapers.

Eighteen months later we celebrated our second miracle, the birth of our son, Philip Mark Read.

I wrote while the boys napped, interviewing by phone with people I knew, our pediatrician, the minister who married us, the football star neighbor, etc., etc. Bill mailed the stories to the newspapers in time to meet the deadlines.

We were still trying to catch up with left-over medical bills, but we were glad to have a family life, and we were optimistic about our future, as our life calmed down.

Even though I didn't feel ready for a full-time job because the boys were so young, I was recruited a few years later for a job as a writer in the Duke News Bureau and public relations office. In their determination to hire me they offered all kinds of concessions, such things as times when I might have to be out, to make it a manageable job for a mother. The income made it possible for us to move to a larger apartment next to the campus so I could walk to work, and reliable baby sitters were available from the nursing school nearby.

In retrospect, I think it was probably the most fulfilling job I ever had.

The entire academic atmosphere nurtured my soul. Interviewing and writing stories about famous professors with such brilliant minds, as well as visiting dignitaries, was awesome work. I covered cultural events (part of my beat) with visiting artists, a perk Bill enjoyed with me. I sometimes subbed for our medical writer satisfying my prior interest in that world.

There was a special friendship among the small group of writers and from our desks we could enjoy the view of what is probably the most picturesque campus anywhere. The lush greenery and flowering bushes in the stillness of southern air provided a long season to enjoy nature's display.

Words flowed easily in that atmosphere.

After a couple of years we made a decision to move to Bill's native New Jersey, partly because we did not agree with the attitudes of many southerners and didn't want our sons to grow up there. Some of their toddler companions were already becoming "rednecks."

Bill still remembered his experience when he first came to Duke at the age of seventeen and gave his seat on a bus to a pregnant black woman. The other passengers jeered him and the bus driver physically put him off the bus, with threats.

Later, Bill worked with the first Afro-American chemist at the Durham water plant and they became friends. Bill visited him at his home, and when word got back to his boss Bill was warned that he had put his job in jeopardy.

I felt deprived because I had no opportunity to meet Afro-Americans, other than to say "hello" to associates' "cleaning ladies," whose pay was so low that they were often employed by people barely above the poverty level themselves. That was life in the South.

It was a time before integration became law. Native southerners were adamant as black citizens began to demand their rights—and they were afraid of each other. The roots of the civil rights movement were beginning as we were moving north.

There were many adjustments to be made in our new life in New Jersey and in some ways it was like starting all over again.

Apartments were harder to find in the area we needed, and more expensive than in the south, the cooler climate had to be adjusted to after those years in the sultry south without air conditioning, the fast pace of life of everyone after the leisurely attitude of southerners, the 24-hour noise of traffic and planes flying overhead—all added up to a new life style.

We discovered that with shopping available every day, all day and at all hours made it easy to find whatever we needed. Anything we couldn't find in New Jersey must not exist. We discovered the New Jersey had everything, including a drive in movie where we could take our little boys in their PJ's.

Just after we settled in our garden apartment in Hackensack and I had begun my search for a job in New York, the boys got the measles—and I caught them.

Bill was already settling into his job as senior chemist at the Passaic Valley Water Commission in Little Falls, N.J. with his typical scientific dedication and passion. He had set up interviews by mail and phone prior to our moving to New Jersey.

He chose not to accept corporate opportunities to opt for a more fulfilling work environment. Bill's jobs had never been about personal ambitions but about being the best at what he was pursuing.

Now it was all about the safety of the drinking water and the millions of people who depended on it. He always kept up with everything new in the field through new editions of textbooks and environmental publications and research. His pursuit inspired other PVWC employees to call him "the professor."

Bill was an environmentalist, always reminding me to be careful with household chemicals. He took extra care with lawn and swimming pool chemicals, eliminating them when possible.

At work, he persevered when he was investigating ways to improve the water quality, testifying in court against the polluters he had uncovered, or any of the other responsibilities that made up his working life. He never considered being "on call" an intrusion because he respected being "a public servant." A man of integrity, Bill always believed in doing "the right thing."

My career path in our new life was slower to materialize.

The first job I had in Manhattan was too comfortable. It was so comfortable that some of the other copywriters in the advertising department of the publishing company had been there for ten years, still with low pay and no place to advance.

Our workplace was one giant room with a center core of cubicles for copywriters, with the husband and wife art team by the one big window for the natural light they needed. Along the other walls were the office staff and one private office for the vice president whom I remember as a nice middle-age man who smiled and said good morning and then disappeared for "wherever."

On Monday morning each of us copywriters received a sheet with the ad copy and book jacket copy assignments and layouts for the technical and academic books of the house for the week. I had only been there about a month when I had all of my week's assignments finished by Wednesday, and didn't know what to do with the down time. I liked the geniality of the work place, and our frequent lunches at a nearby armory where the servers were war veterans and the food was good and inexpensive. The other copywriters were all native New Yorkers from boroughs like Queens and Brooklyn and were nicely different from the driven ambitious out-of-towners that I would later meet in Manhattan. It was a laid-back job that didn't meet my salary needs—or ambitions.

My urgent need for a better salary to cover commuting and child care expenses, with something left over, took me back to The New York Times ads and a job as a technical editor for the trade association for the petroleum industry. The salary was much higher and the office overlooked the Rockefeller Plaza skating rink which was especially scenic when the giant Christmas tree was there. But the job proved to be boring and lonely. My two "roommates" were also native New Yorkers but not friendly, and I think they considered me an intruder. The head of the division was a middle aged "Texas gal" complete with drawl and a flirting nature that took her out of our office most of the time as she roamed the other three floors of the association where the Texas men were. I didn't want to waste my working life there.

Pursuing the Times ads for a third time, I came across an ad seeking "a good writer interested in public relations"—but it was in New Jersey. It intrigued me because it sounded like an entrepreneurial opportunity, and after meeting with the one-man operation, I decided to take the challenge and give it a try.

When we started working together, typing our own press releases and pursuing new business from a tiny office in Clifton, New Jersey we began to grow with small accounts. As former journalists we worked well together as we struggled to become incorporated as an agency, Public Relations Counsel, Inc.

The breakthrough came with the acquisition of our first Johnson & Johnson account enabling us to move our office to Manhattan. We were on our way.

Our first New York office was at 18 East 41st Street. Our short block ended at the New York Public Library with the big lions guarding the entrance. I loved those lions, especially at Christmas when they were adorned with wreaths around their necks. Our employees gave me replicas of them: bookends that I decorate with tiny wreaths every Christmas.

The building was old and small and our suite was the former office of the building owner which left us with the benefits of a bathroom, a kitchen and other amenities befitting a public relations agency.

The only other office on our floor belonged to a well-known literary agent, Annie Laurie Williams, who represented Harper Lee's "To Kill a Mocking Bird," and other best-seller authors.

Annie was a nice little lady that I thought of as old, who made a habit of introducing me to famous authors when we were on the elevator as "Glory is a writer too." The flattery prompted me to start the book that I never finished. Annie kept urging me to continue because the subject of combining career and family was a new "hot" topic at the time, but I was too busy living it to have the time to write it.

In only a few years, the agency grew to a staff of twelve with an impressive roster of corporations as clients—and continued to grow. Our Johnson & Johnson clients stayed with us for the life of the agency, and I learned respect for some corporations from this ethical company.

A meeting at J & J headquarters was like a vacation day. The employees called the new building "the love boat," and it was wonderfully unlike most corporate headquarters.

When I walked into the reception area, it was like a magnificent garden room with luxurious sofas and chairs and oriental rugs, all surrounded by trees in pots that were tended by gardeners. Skylights bathed the area in natural light.

The offices were off the circular walkway above that looked down on the huge reception area, resembling an ocean liner.

I frequently ran into the CEO in the reception area, and he always thanked me for "the wonderful public relations support you are providing for our brands." It was an ego trip to be able to feel that our efforts were appreciated. In public relations, it's typical to get "static" from clients who often demand "miracles."

In a few years another sudden change, typical of my life, surfaced. We had just moved into our house in Clifton, N.J. the reality of our long ago dream. I was sitting on the living room floor happily sorting things when the phone rang with the startling news of the accidental death of my business partner and friend, at the age of thirty-six. It was an unexpected blow that added to my sadness.

My planned time off for settling into our new home was cancelled, and ahead of me was the responsibility of keeping the agency going.

It required more working time because it added more business responsibilities to my creative concentration that had been my primary job as vice president.

Bill's belief in my abilities and his encouragement with "everything will be all right" gave me determination. "You can do it," he kept telling me.

I had already learned that the only choice is to go on—but death always seemed to be intruding on the progress of our life.

As I took over as president and stabilized the agency, things were hectic but rewarding. Every day was different and unpredictable. Some

were exciting and some were glamorous, and all of them were antici-
pated with wonder as I rode my commuter bus to my office.

Many of my days were filled with lunches with editors at Sardie's
where celebrities sat by walls covered with caricatures and signed pictures of other celebrities. Other lunches were at restaurants like The
Russian Tea Room, restaurants in The Pierre and The Plaza, steak row
restaurants, and the little French places favored by editors of fashion
and the like magazines.

A more personal aspect of lunching was with Burt Bacharach. He
frequently greeted me with, "wait till you hear what the kids are up to
now." The syndicated columnist was referring to his musician son of
the same name and his daughter-in-law Angie Dickinson. He had
introduced them and never tired of talking about their lives.

There were trips to San Francisco where I met Tony Bennett, to
frigid Chicago, to torrid Dallas, to New Orleans before the flood, and
all the major cities of the United States, and to some of the "boonies" as
well. It was a travel education.

There were trips to clients' national sales meetings where I usually
made three presentations a day to acquaint the sales executives with the
great public relations support they were receiving. These were resort
areas, such as Paradise Island in the Bahamas; all my arrangements had
been made for me.

The grand opening of a client restaurant, The Jade Fountain, in
Paramus, N.J. was the big dream of three enterprising young men who
had built the upscale Chinese restaurant. We made the event a benefit
for the cancer society, to introduce the New York and New Jersey food
and entertainment media, and the future clientele, to the new metropolitan area hot spot.

Bill's old neighbors kept popping up whenever we were in Bergen
County and this opening was no exception. When someone shouted,

"Bill Read," he recognized one of his old high school girl friends who was there as a representative of the cancer society.

This was our introduction to gourmet Chinese food that made addicts of our whole family. Our love of Chinese food continued even after Bill died, when son Bill and I lunched on our "soul food" as we spent time together that helped save me from despair. It was typical to find myself in unusual places, like Yogi Berra's yard watching the excavation for the installation of a Buster Crabbe swimming pool for our client. It was PR action with photographers shooting the pictures for the full-page story that appeared in The New York Daily News. At another time, I was walking down a Manhattan street with Buster Crabbe when he was accosted by autograph seekers, even though it had been years since he was "Tarzan."

Bill and I were invited by a magazine editor to the opening of a hip new night club, "Cheetah." We shared the fun of being at this psychedelic-like event with a flashing revolving ball over the raised stage, loud music, and celebrities everywhere.

There were always client meetings and all kinds of writing to do, press releases, pamphlets, feature stories, film scripts, and speeches for clients to add the warm personal touch to their notes.

New business presentations were more daunting now because my business partner and I had perfected a good team, doing our homework and using a cue system that came across as knowledgeable and creative. Our demeanor from our reporting background added to the sincerity of our "pitch." My woman's approach had been important, but now there were prospective clients who felt the need for a male presence. My later accounts were often from referrals from clients who knew of my work for Johnson & Johnson.

Press parties, trade shows, seminars, etc. were often accompanied by social events with star entertainment, often from running Broadway shows. Bill enjoyed these evenings with me as my admired escort with a friendly demeanor. I particularly remember one night when we were in a hotel elevator on the way to the top floor for a dinner dance gala to honor journalists. He struck up a conversation with our elevator companion by commenting, "This should be a wonderful evening," and she responded to the gentlemanly warmth in his voice, continuing the conversation until we entered the ballroom. She turned out to be the honored recipient of a top newspaper award. Bill always made friends wherever we went, including the movie stars and other celebrities we encountered in the course of my career.

The necessity to "dress for success" was an additional burden of my job because I wasn't really into fashion except for my attraction to glamorous evening gowns. I was privy to some seventh-avenue show rooms where I could sometimes purchase sample clothing—and there was always Loehman's. Women wore suits to work.

I still have a closet full of vintage clothes from the sixties and seventies, and well-worn high-heel shoes that walked me all over Manhattan, before someone found the obvious answer for the torture. Later, it became fashionable to wear sneakers from place to place whenever it was possible to change when you reached your destination.

When Bill asked me, "Where is my red tie?" or "Have you seen my cuff links?", he reflected his father's "gentlemanly" fashion sense. The platinum cuff links were an inheritance from his grandfather and Bill had a strong sense of family lineage. As an alternative to suits, men could wear gray pants, and a Navy blue blazer with a white shirt and a tie.

Bill still wanted to bestow gifts on me that had not been possible earlier in our lives, which lead to the acquisition of a long black mink coat that he insisted on buying for me for about $3,000 at the Flemington N.J. Fur Company.

At the time I was frequently appearing on Joan Fontaine's early cable television show on behalf of my clients, and we became friendly. The show was taped in an area of the Bronx where no cab would venture, so I rode to and back to Manhattan with her in her limo. Joan was in a designer fur company ad that featured famous actresses who were legends wearing mink coats worth at least $100,000. One day Joan commented, "Oh, we have the same coat." They looked the same to me too.

It was a challenging but interesting time to be a career woman in New York. Women had not gained much equality, and I often found myself as the only woman in a group of men in such places as the delegates' dining room at the United Nations, Gracie Mansion, and the Overseas Press Club, as well as other male dominated lunches and meetings. I remember a luncheon that I had arranged for a client at the Yale (University) Club and secured Mayor John Lindsay to be the speaker. No women were allowed at the club, and it took "Yalie" John Lindsay himself to get me in.

Although I supported the women's liberation movement and carried a membership card, I had a few issues with some of the aspects. I always believed in family life and being a woman was just one of the other obstacles to overcome in my career path. Advancements in the cause have helped everyone, but equality will truly arrive when all women get equal pay—and we elect a woman as president of the United States. I advise my granddaughters to avoid the left-over "macho" guys and look for the males who "make you fell good about yourself and respect your ambitions."

Bill never had any bias against women pursuing their ambitions, and he was always supportive of the women in his work place. He was proud of my career, and his appreciation was inspiring for me. He made me feel like I could do anything.

I had my share of trying experiences at work, but I was fortunate to have some clients and bosses with enlightened attitudes too.

Our family life stayed close to home because the demands of being president of the agency made it difficult to plan many real family vacations other than our short ones to the Jersey shore. However, we did manage to have two enriching trips.

Fortunately, Bill and I never had wanderlust after his travel time in the Navy, and my nomadic childhood and regular business trips. We had already sent Bill and Phil alone on their first airplane trip to San Francisco to visit their Aunt Jan and Uncle Jack and cousins, Jackie and Jeremy.

Our trip to London and Paris originated because my staff was always pointing out to me that I had never been abroad, and it dawned on me that our upcoming twentieth wedding anniversary would be an ideal time for our big trip, now that the agency was under control and our sons were in high school.

When I asked Bill how he would feel about a trip to London and Paris in celebration of our anniversary, he said, "Are you kidding?", with a surprised look on his face, and added, "Can we do it?" The boys' reactions were similar.

Bill's ancestors were from England and neither of us had been there so all the wonders of that great city were exciting, but the friendliness of the "Brits" was what we enjoyed most. We stayed in the ancient Hotel Russell with few amenities, except for the hotel's pub frequented by natives. Bill and I spent many happy hours there, drinking beer and talking, and making friends, who gave us the real flavor of the city. Bill and Phil were off to Carnaby Street which was at the height of the Beatles era and their favorite haunt.

In Paris we stayed at the old traditionally elegant Hotel Scribe with crystal chandeliers and gold everywhere. We dined in the Eiffel Tower restaurant with its breathtaking view of that beautiful city at night, but the maitre d' expressed his dislike for our long-haired sons and the floor show got risqué enough that we decided to leave early.

On an extremely warm Easter Sunday, we took the tourist boat ride down the Seine and we all got sunburned. We convinced our sons to go with us to our favorite opera, "Madame Butterfly" but they left early. We took in everything, all the famous sights, and spent hours in the Louvre.

After sightseeing, Bill and I drank wine in the sidewalk cafes, and talked at length without distractions like we used to. Bill and Phil abandoned us to test their high school French to get cab drivers to take them to Montmarte, where I suspect they may have drunk some wine. After all, they were artists "hanging out" at that famous place.

We flew home on a new giant 747 that had just come out, to end our big family vacation that has been long remembered by all of us and stands out as the best of our sojourns.

Another travel highlight for Bill and I was my twenty-fifth Duke class reunion which was a sentimental journey with intense ties to the place where we began our life together.

Revisiting the campus, with the new buildings of its growth, was the same in its difference. The Gothic architecture preserved the remembered atmosphere, as we spotted old familiar places where so many years ago we sat and talked about our future.

"Do you remember those steps?" Bill asked with a smile.

"Of course, how could I not remember?" I replied.

"That's where I first told you that I would always love you and we would always be together and gave you my fraternity pin," he said.

We reminisced with old friends, particularly with those who like us had college romances that became long marriages, as we shared our life stories. At the big gala of the weekend the romantic music of our era inspired us to remember the wonder of those times. Bill kept commenting "It's so wonderful to be here again with you."

Only a few of the women from my class had careers and in my difference was a kind of "fame." A few years earlier, I had returned to the campus to be on a communication career panel, which had been a thrill for me as well.

As a lark, I unsuccessfully looked for a girl that I was in awe of during my freshman year. She was from Upper Montclair, N.J.—a place I had never heard of then but where I have since spent a lot of time. She was a beauty queen and a top student and I thought of her as the epitome of someone who must have a perfect life.

The city of Durham was not so familiar because of its growth as a result of the Research Triangle, which brought new people and companies to the academic center. We had previously taken our sons on a summer trip to show them where they lived before they started school in New Jersey.

When Bill and I went to the Duke reunion we were in the highlight period of our life with a family and a comfortable life style. By our standards, we had it all.

The reunion was the only college one we ever attended, and I never went to any of my high school reunions. We did go to Bill's twentieth Bogota, New Jersey high school reunion which was rewarding for me to meet his old friends, who told him, "You look the same." One of his old girlfriends, on her second husband, wanted us to get together socially, but we never pursued it.

After the Duke reunion, which was as much Bill's as mine, he said, "We'll go back for our fiftieth."

Life, however, has a way of interfering with plans.

Sometimes the realization of the time for a career change comes slowly and requires a lot of soul searching. It's a little "scary" too.

After more than twenty-five years of commuting to Manhattan and the fast-track work style, my lease in the Helmsley Building expiring (with the rent to double), along with the "burn out" I had begun to experience forced me to think about and explore a change.

An offer from a corporate client for an internal public relations job tempted me greatly but it would have been an impossible commute to south Jersey. I reluctantly had to turn it down. A giant international advertising agency offered me a job in their PR division but I couldn't see myself in that atmosphere—and I knew that what they really wanted was for me to bring my accounts to them. A west coast agency wanted to merge but that was no temptation for me.

My frustrations of working in New York communications had by now overshadowed the glamour and excitement. The thrill was gone. And I was tired.

There was so much to deal with, in addition to the work itself.

The down side of blackouts and trying to walk to Port Authority bus terminal in the dark for buses that weren't running, the garbage strikes and walking around the stench from the sidewalk blocked with garbage from the restaurant next door, being offered drugs while walking past Bryant Park, spending hours in hot summer in a non-air conditioned bus stuck in the Lincoln Tunnel, were exhausting. Seeing beautiful teenagers everywhere "stoned," and the media people who abused alcohol with three martini lunches that often stretched into the cocktail hour were discouraging sights.

In addition to the usual hassles, New York is also full of perils, and I had my share.

My first experience was at noontime in a restaurant where I was meeting an editor for lunch. The entrance was dimly lit and a step caused me to trip and fall, breaking my ankle. The only thing the restaurant did was bring me a drink. My ankle was in a cast to my knee for several weeks. Bill had to drive me into the city and pick me up which was important to my lawsuit. However, the attorney recommended a settlement and by the time he took his percentage, I became the looser.

My second episode was when my wallet was lifted cleverly and swiftly from my pocketbook when I was in a bookstore. I immediately became aware of what happened, and loudly said "someone help me." The proprietor rushed me right out of the store. I saw a policeman, but his only response was to point in a direction saying, "the precinct is that way." When I found the station, the unfriendly officer gave me his spiel. "Lady this is New York, this happens dozens of times every day. There's nothing we can do. The thief usually takes the cash and throws the wallet into a mailbox. When this happens, we'll call you." And it happened as he said. Because I had no money, I had to walk many blocks to Port Authority bus terminal, where the traveler's aide office gave me a pass so I could get home.

The most unbelievable and devastating event was when I was accused of shoplifting. It was such a bad experience that I returned to my office in tears to be consoled by my employees.

In a drug store near my office, I was approached by a security person who asked me "Where did you put it?"

I said, "What?"

"The lipstick you stole," he replied.

I was so shocked that I offered to take everything out of my pocketbook and my pockets to prove my innocence. He called the store manager, who started shouting at me in an abusive manner. I emptied my pocketbook and took off my coat. He threw both on the floor, and became so violently enraged that the security man had to restrain him, and said to me, "You better leave the store before he hurts you." When I told the policeman out on the street he basically ignored me.

I wrote a letter (some of my best writing) to the president of the chain that bore his name. He never responded. I should have sued, even though the lawyer didn't think I had a case without witnesses.

Everyone who has worked in Manhattan has tales to tell.

The time for change had come and even though there was some apprehension I could bravely walk away without regrets. The history of my agency is in eight big file cabinets in my basement, stuffed with the vast information that public relations amass.

Working in public relations is an education like going to graduate school in many areas. It's an opportunity to witness all sides of life and meet all kinds of people—and it raises awareness of how alike we all are, even in our differences. It's the upside of a career that often gets a "bad rap."

The new life style was a big adjustment as I closed my agency and moved into freelance writing again, but it provided more free time to enjoy things that had been hard to fit into such a hectic life. Bill and I savored the quiet experiences that we missed because there had always been so many responsibilities, so many adjustments, and so much of everything demanding our immediate attention. We were able to spend more time together than we had since college days. We went back to being the couple we were when we concentrated on each other. We went to all the dinner dances of Bill's numerous professional affiliations and became dancing partners again. Bill kept saying, "We have such a good life."

Our sons had graduated from college and married and were having children of their own, and now we had time to enjoy being grandparents.

Grandparenthood provided a second chance to renew and experience the wonder of watching those we love during the early part of their lives.

While some memories of our own sons are crystal clear, some of the actual physical feelings had become a little faded by time. To once again experience the feeling of warmth from a baby's arms wrapped around your neck, to see the incredible smile of pure innocence, and to hear the joyful "giggles" is a sweet promise of life going on.

We had a chance to relive the magic and the plus of learning about "little girls" through our three granddaughters led by our first grandchild Lauren, as our lone grandson Philip Jr. continued the male dominant line. We had it all again, soccer and basketball games, dance recitals, first communions, proms, graduations, and all the other events and rites of passage.

Bill summed it up with, "We are so fortunate to see our children have children."

Now there was opportunity for neglected projects as well so faced with unfamiliar leisure time, I decide to "down size" all the stuff that had accumulated all around the house. The daunting project uncovered nostalgic things that had been forgotten, even though it didn't come up with some of the things that I had previously tried to find. Bill and I laughed when we came across old college essays, cards and invitations, our love notes, and things significant of earlier times like World War II ration books and a copy of Life magazine with Marilyn Monroe on the cover. When I had only thrown away a few scraps of paper, I realized that I couldn't toss these treasures, so that ended the project. It was too much like throwing away a part of us.

Anyway, there were obvious reminders of our life in plain view. The baby grand piano in the family room is a reminder of its acquisition while I was on a business trip. Bill and the boys were shopping at a music store, when Bill saw the used McPhail of Boston piano and evidently felt a need to own it. With the boys urging him to buy "the real bargain," the deal was closed, and was the surprise of my return home. None of us could really play the piano, but they considered it a treasure they had uncovered. Returning home to son Bill's pierced ear (a big deal in those days) was another surprise. My son said, "Dad thinks it's okay," and his father said, "I didn't think you would mind." There are reminders in our basement of the high school jamming sessions that brought the police a few times with a request to bring it down a decibel. There is an antique amplifier that Bill built from a Heath Kit still there, but the drums and electric guitar have moved on. The pool table is still used by the grandchildren, who may be "sharks."

Other benefits of our new life emerged as well.

The Jersey shore was always beckoning. It was our favorite place, and now we could go there more often.

Bill and I loved walking along the ocean edge holding hands and quietly enjoying the déjà vu, going all the way back to the college Spring break at Myrtle Beach, South Carolina.

Entranced by the crisp air of an early summer morning, with the warm sand tickling our toes and the cool water splashing against our legs, we listened to the soothing gentle ocean roar that shuts out the world.

"This is the life," Bill always said. And I agreed with him even though I can't swim and am, in fact, afraid of the water but that doesn't keep me from appreciating the lure of the seashore and how it can push away life's cares.

When we were there with family members, first our sons and later with their wives and our grandchildren as well, Bill joined them swimming and playing in the water while I watched them from under an umbrella with contentment and peace. Later, we would enjoy lobster and shrimp at the Lobster Shanty at Point Pleasant or maybe out on the pier. I can still taste those meals.

Bill loved the water, the ocean and our swimming pool.

Every morning before he treated the pool water, he swam his few laps, and then we would leisurely sit on the deck and gaze at the sparkling azure of the pool surrounded by lush greenery to enjoy the peaceful feeling. The pool was ready for whatever group might be swimming that day.

The more leisurely life in the suburbs was an enjoyable and calming period we needed, even though we did not know what was ahead.

It was only a few years respite of rewarding family life before another life chapter—more challenging and profound—erupted.

It would be the ultimate test of Bill's "everything will be all right" philosophy.

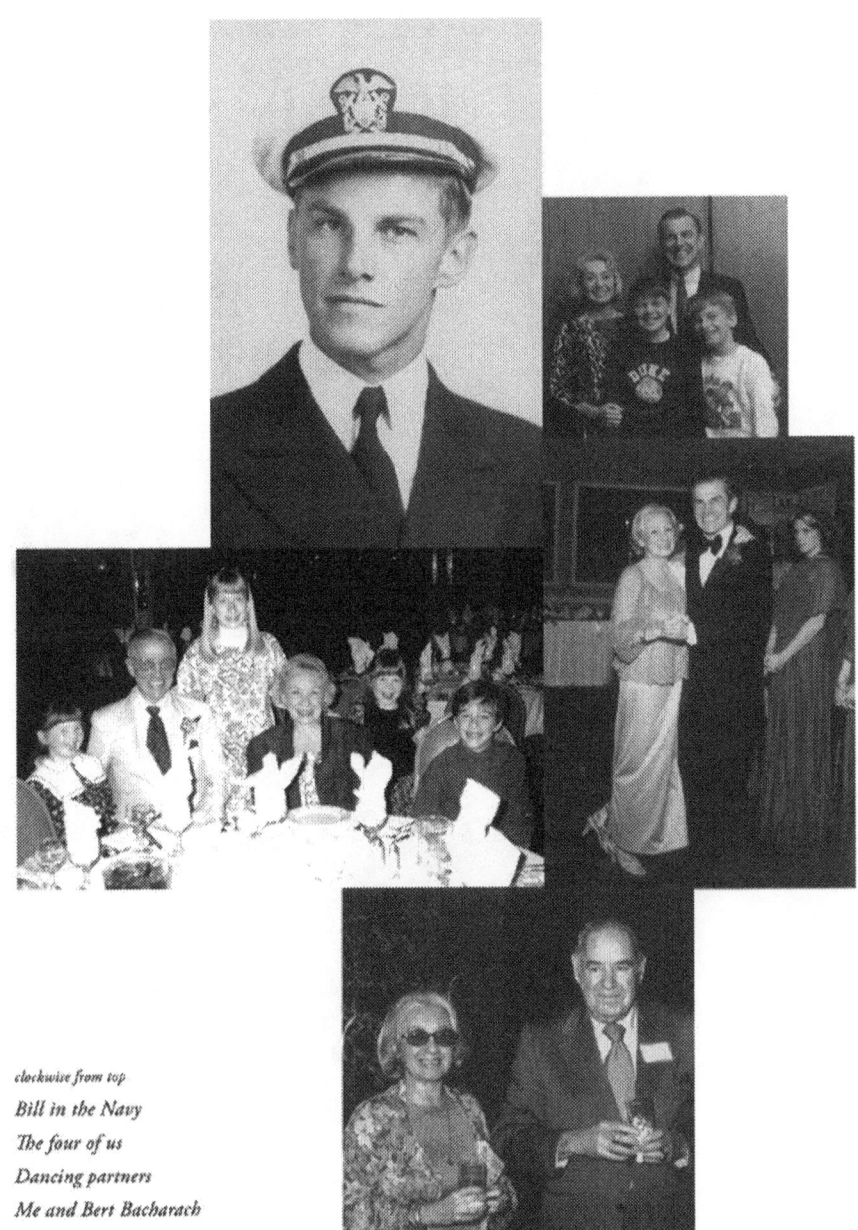

clockwise from top
Bill in the Navy
The four of us
Dancing partners
Me and Bert Bacharach
Bill's retirement dinner

clockwise from top
**Grandchildren
Christmas 2006**
Bill and Glory
Our family
**By the pool with
Leanna and Keirsten**

PART IV
Along Came Alzheimer's

As I lay on the gurney in the hospital corridor waiting for the X-rays of my broken wrist after falling down the basement steps, and medication for the pain that distracted me, I wondered where Bill was. He had disappeared.

When I had arrived at the emergency room with my dangling hand, described by my doctor as, "The worst I have ever seen," Bill went to call our sons. I later learned that he had called them, saying I "was fine"—then got lost in the hospital.

He wandered around the hospital looking for me and didn't reappear until hours later, just before I went into the operating room. He said, "I couldn't find you."

The next day when I was told I could go home, he was missing again. My call to our home was unanswered and he wasn't with either of the boys. I found him at his office and he seemed normal, although not aware of his totally out of character behavior of the previous day, or that day.

When I told our family physician about Bill's behavior, he gave him the mini mental test that is the first of many tests that lead to a possible diagnosis of Alzheimer's. The test is simple, such as hearing a small group of words to memorize, a simple arithmetic problem, and questions like, "Who is the president of the United States?" Bill probably scored a D.

With typical compassion in his voice, our doctor told me that he suspected Alzheimer's and that there is no cure for the fatal disease, but it didn't sink in that day.

He recommended a cat scan to begin the process of eliminating other possible causes of dementia, such as mini strokes, that impair memory and logical thinking. Bill's scan was negative.

The next step was an evaluation at a health center. This was an all-day event with doctors of various specialties testing him physically and psychologically, while psychologists and social workers talked endlessly with me about his entire life, filling up pages of information. Then he had an MRI.

The conclusion was possible Alzheimer's.

It wasn't long before Bill admitted to me that he was having problems remembering. A scientist and a former World War II naval officer who was an executive and research director at a municipal water company he couldn't even do simple math now.

The diagnosis of Alzheimer's is usually a surprise because this insidious disease starts before anything seems to be wrong. It only sends out vague clues. It was only in retrospect that I realized that the subtle early signs had been there. Thinking back, I remembered the summer a few years earlier when Bill went back to our alma mater for a summer course in computer programming. He called home every day often complaining "I can't seem to be able to do the work." I told him to talk to the professor, not thinking that anything was wrong.

The word "Alzheimer's" had not been mentioned to Bill and the possibility went right by him, but I had already begun to worry even though I knew very little about the disease at the time. Although I did not tell him then, I began to research the disease and soon amassed a drawer full of Alzheimer's literature.

With each book, pamphlet and article my fears grew. In my heart and mind, I knew that we were embarking on the saddest journey of our lives.

Although I believed he had a right to know, it was hard to find the courage to tell him but I was so distressed that I could no longer keep to myself what I knew was as close to a diagnosis as possible.

The day I told Bill he had Alzheimer's we clung to each other and wept. Neither of us had ever been criers, but this was one of the most profound moments of our life. We knew we were in this together and it would take both of us to keep this disease from robbing us of our time together. Our marriage was a partnership and our commitment was to face everything in life together. We would share his disease was my silent vow.

After Bill's diagnosis, there were important practical things that had to be quickly resolved before we could continue with our life.

When Bill came home from work and started expressing difficulty in doing his job up to his standards, it seemed to be the time for him to retire even though that had not been in our plans before.

The solution presented itself with a special retirement package that I encouraged him to take and along with his own frustration at work this early transition—one of many that I would have to orchestrate—moved us into a new life style.

Driving a car is something else that has to be stopped early in the disease because lapses of attention and reasoning begin early on. It's a difficult transition because cars are so closely associated with independence. Bill is usually cooperative but he resisted this request and it took our doctor's tactful words and my dire assessment of the condition of the older car he had been driving, after losing his company car, to convince him. He complained for a while when I became our chauffeur, and then forgot about it. I was already discovering that forgetting becomes an ally when dealing with Alzheimer's.

Now that these frustrating decisions were out of the way, Bill and I were able to become a little more relaxed.

We often sat on our deck and gazed at the now defunct swimming pool, allegedly closed for repairs but really for his safety, and reminisced about the pool parties and the fun it provided for our sons and their friends, and later our grandchildren. It had often been commented that Bill kept the water so pure that you could drink it.

Bill was still the friendly person everyone knew and it was not obvious that he had Alzheimer's. His smile was like sunshine on a dreary day and he had a sense of humor. One fall day he was trying to rake leaves when a motorist topped to ask directions. Bill smiled, and logically said, "I'm sorry but you better ask someone else because I have Alzheimer's."

Bill's Alzheimer's was slowly moving along but not in any scheduled way and he was not especially distressed about his difficulty with simple things unless it was something of particular importance to him. He couldn't tie his tie and that did bother him because he always wore a tie, even when he mowed the lawn.

He was constantly losing things. Our granddaughter Leanna found his first missing wallet in the pocket of the pool table, and then he lost it for the last time elsewhere.

Alzheimer's progresses slowly, with surprising outbreaks and calm periods, but it is erratic—and varies with individuals. Even when awareness seems intact, fatigue can be a part of the disease.

Bill's visit to the old-fashioned barber shop he had gone to for years was an indicator of his disease's physical progress, I helped him into the chair and he and the barber chatted about their families, but when I tried to get him out of the chair, it took help from a strong young man who was waiting for his turn to get Bill to his feet.

We tried the drugs that were supposed to help symptoms or slow down the disease, but they didn't help Bill. Looking for a cure should be the goal, and maybe the answer is in stem cell research.

During this early part of the disease, we tried to do all the things we had been doing in recent years and settled into a routine. Bill would ask, "Where are we going today?" We went to the concerts in Brookdale Park for the big band music of our college days and the Fourth of July fireworks, we went to flea markets and street fairs, we went to art shows and dined out. When his ability to make decisions waned, Bill would lean on me, telling the waitress in a restaurant, "I'll have what my wife is having."

He was physically well and cognizant enough for us to socialize and shop. In the supermarket, he told all the young mothers, "You have a beautiful child." He made their day for all the people he encountered. He was taking an art class at the high school two days a week and seemed to enjoy it even though he had lost the talent he once had, but he became friends with the instructor. Making friends was a talent that he never lost. He did an oil portrait of me many years ago that I treasure now more than ever.

Every day I would have little excursions planned to get us out of the house into the big world.

Part of our daily rituals was to have a glass of wine and salad around 4 PM and our dinner about 5 PM before his fatigue caught up with him. As his awareness waned and his lethargy increased, we gradually had to eliminate some of those things.

He liked to watch "Jeopardy" and surprised me on several occasions by knowing the answer to some obscure question that the contestants missed. Bill's memory had always been superior to mine. He remembered old phone numbers and the exact times of our meeting, pin up, etc. I didn't remember the details of these events.

He tried to do the things he had always done. He tried to mow the lawn and do home repairs, but I soon had to distract him for his own safety. He tired to vacuum and do laundry but they usually had to be done over. The last chore that he hung on to was taking the garbage can to the curb. He would get halfway there and go back. He just couldn't remember how to do these things. My heart cried as I watched him struggling to hold on to his independence.

In early disease, I became acutely aware of the important role our home played in the "in sickness" part of our life. Being with me in our haven helped him to weather this harsh disease with dignity and love.

One day as we sat on the living room couch, the late day sun illuminated the dining room through the sliding glass doors to the deck that Bill had built. The sun moved around toward its destination in the west. It glowed outside the glass and imparted and enchanting surrealist view of the dining room and the trees beyond. The aroma of the lilacs from our yard enhanced the mood.

We looked, and Bill said, "We have a nice home, don't we?", but it wasn't a question. It was a special time of the day when we savored the serenity of being together in our haven with one of those elusive feelings of appreciation that make life so worthwhile.

From our living room couch, we quietly viewed the rosy glow of the day's end through the big picture window.

I reminisced about the acquisition of each piece of furniture and decoration and he listened. Everything has a story. Bill didn't remember, but when I told him he smiled. I knew he shared the feeling with me even though it was fleeting.

As the eerie shadows approached, his fatigue took him. We retired and he slept peacefully by my side. Sleep evaded me, but even as I reviewed the trials of that Alzheimer's day I appreciated having him with me.

The next morning, the early sun glowed in the butter-yellow kitchen as Bill slowly descended the few stairs and said, "There you are." We silently looked at our gallery wall of favorite family photos.

We often took coffee to our deck to watch the early morning sun glisten on the twin towers of the World Trade Center. It was only six months after Bill's death that I watched the smoky haze of 9/11 from our deck. On that historically tragic day, our grandson Philip Mark, Jr. was in his dorm at the School of Visual Arts in lower Manhattan, and his parents had difficulty getting him out of New York and safely home to New Jersey.

Our home held importance for me because my childhood had not been spent in "homey" abodes. Depending on my family's financial situation, my nomadic childhood had been spent in boarding houses, hotels and motels until we acquired a luxury trailer. I had fantasized about living in a real house with a room of my own that would become a permanent home—a dream that prevailed throughout my childhood and beyond my adolescence.

During the years my mother was in the tuberculosis sanitarium, I lived with my Aunt Jo who had saved me from the orphanage. When my Mom and Dad were with me again we lived in three rooms in part of a house. There was no central heat or hot water, we shared a bathroom with another family, and I slept on the living room couch.

A number of years passed before Bill and I lived in our "dream home." But, when we did, I fell so hopelessly in love with our suburban split level that I didn't even feel a tinge of envy when in the course of my career I had visited the habitats of celebrities. Not even Joan Bennett's penthouse overlooking Central Park, or Arlene Dahl's big house high up in the sky that looked like an elegant suburban mansion, elevated in the sky to provide a panoramic view.

Recalling my business trips, I realize that I never appreciated the grand hotels—not even San Francisco's Fairmont or Boston's Copley Plaza, because I was anxious to return home.

Our home embraced us when we needed it. It is a diary of our life and now I am the keeper of these memories. I could never live any place else.

Bill was always sensitive to my special feelings about our home, and he grew to share them as our life moved on, often repeating, "We have a nice home, don't we?"

Although roaming is typical of people with Alzheimer's, Bill never really strayed, which I think is because of his strong attachment to our home. However, he did give me a scare in mid-disease when I was still involved as a trustee of St. Peter's Haven, a homeless family shelter and food pantry in Clifton when it was still supposed to be safe to leave him alone for short periods. I went to a short meeting and when I went to the car to return home there he was trying to load his bike into the trunk. He had ridden on busy streets, and gave me my first big scare for his safety. He had remembered how to get there to my amazement. Needless to say, he was never home alone again.

A short time later he got lost at the mall. I turned in another direction for a minute—and he was gone. My heart began racing, I notified security and started running around looking for him. Finally, I found him in the parking lot sitting on the hood of our car. He was smiling and not distressed as he asked, "Where were you?" He thought that I was the one who was lost.

Another mall incident was when he went into the bathroom and couldn't find his way out. Waiting outside, I was becoming nervous when Bill came out with a kind young man who had rescued him. Bill thanked him and so did I, and it made me feel better to know that there are caring people around who probably don't realize what they have done for you.

Seeking help with my own stress, I went to my first Alzheimer's support meeting with apprehension, but I needed to find ways to deal with our life as it was becoming. I thought I would never return but I did. It not only helped me cope as things became more difficult but gave me strength to go on living the one-day-at-a-time philosophy. Relating to people in similar situations makes it easier.

Bonding with fellow travelers in the group was especially helpful because they were the people who could truly understand. Some of them were in denial and searched the world for a cure, but most of us accepted the disease and were determined to do the best we could to keep as much quality of life possible. We got compassion and emotional strength from each other.

The support meetings often had a speaker who was a doctor, lawyer or social worker. While they were informative, they can also add to your worries when a doctor describes how people with Alzheimer's die by choking on food or from starvation. And, attorneys make predictions that the disease will leave you destitute unless you are wealthy, and social workers recommend an entire overhaul of your home. As a practical person I heeded some of their advice but I discovered that if you don't panic and make use of common sense, you will be able to solve these problems as they come along. Alzheimer's is a long disease.

Fatigue and stress began to make life difficult as I piled guilt on myself for things I couldn't control. We were both suffering from this disease that had really just begun and could end in only one way. I became worried and fearful.

When my stress level began to escalate even more, I decided to send Bill to an Alzheimer's day care center program for four hours a day two days a week. He didn't see why he had to go but he went to please me. I drove him there and picked him up and he started complaining while we were riding, so I decided to have the center's bus transport him. This worked better, thanks to the two alternating drivers who treated him with such respect and friendliness that he went willingly for awhile.

But the staff reported to me that once he was there he kept saying "Where is my wife?", "I want to go home," or "I have to call my wife." It was a combination of typical Alzheimer's separation anxiety and his obsession with wanting to be with me all the time. The staff reported that he was friendly and cooperative while there, and he appreciated the young intern who called him her "dancing partner." Women always liked Bill.

One incident at day care stands out in my memory and still makes me feel like crying. After my support meeting, I decided to pick Bill up and went to the center where music was playing. He was quietly sitting at a table, but jumped up when he saw me and quickly came to me crying. I don't have a clue as to what triggered it. I had expected his smile and got it in a few minutes but he was anxious to come home. He recovered quickly, but my sadness lingered for a long time.

A feeling of profound sadness increased as the disease moved along but so did my compassion—and I had the strong feeling of being his protector against Alzheimer's and the world. Alzheimer's was us.

'Emotions far outlive memory' is something I kept learning from Bill.

An invitation to an extended family wedding, prompted me to get out Bill's "Gatsby" suit. The light beige linen and his patterned yellow tie made him look young. When our youngest granddaughter Keirsten asked him to dance, his whole face lit up and made the evening memorable for all of us.

The funeral of the husband of our "best friends" couple is strong evidence too. These were people we shared so much with—husbands were scientists and wives were writers. We had for many years enjoyed all kinds of socializing and they were dear to us. At the church, Bill kept asking, "Who died?" When eulogies were read and our friend's name was mentioned I looked at Bill and saw the tears rolling down his cheeks.

Another event that demonstrated the degree of emotional awareness during the course of this disease was the death of our Irish Setter. Ambie was the sweetest canine girl and Bill's walking companion for years. She became ill and had been in the hospital, but the day she died the whole family visited to comfort her. At bedtime Bill carried her into the living room and laid down on the couch beside her, but during the night he called me because she had peacefully died in her sleep. Bill cried for the loss of his friend. But in a few days the memory was gone. Again, the disease had provided a saving grace.

Even as his disease progressed, we continued to have family dinners for all ten of us on special Sundays and Bill obviously enjoyed being together, but as soon as they all waved good bye, he forgot that they had been here. His emotional memory lasted during the event, but quickly disappeared.

It was not in Bill's nature to complain or be difficult. He appreciated everything in life and it helped him fight his disease.

Our family dinners to celebrate birthdays, anniversaries, and big holidays like Thanksgiving date way back to when we bought our long dining room table shortly after we bought our home. As our family grew so did our table with the extra leaf added so that by the time we reached ten it was just right for us. We each had our own place to sit, with the "baby" of our grandchildren, Keirsten, at one end and Bill at the other.

My desire to be a matriarch had taken me to outlet stores where fine china and table linens for each season could be purchased at a discount price, so the table always looked elegant with flowers of the season. Our crystal chandelier, the pride of my early decorating, was the perfect touch for the dinners.

I often wished I knew how my Mom had perfected her pot roast that lives in my memory. It was plain-food of gourmet quality. When our children were toddlers and our budget was tight, Bill and I practically subsisted on macaroni and cheese and when our sons tasted it they didn't want junior food anymore. Everyone loves mac and cheese.

In spite of a few learning experiences, like the Thanksgiving that we had to call the fire department because the oven was on fire, I perfected my menus and being in the kitchen was a comforting experience, like sitting by a fireplace.

The dinners were more about ambiance than a gourmet menu. They were often prime rib accompanied by "comfort foods" like mashed potatoes and green peas to entice the young grandchildren. Now there are two vegetarians to accommodate with special side dishes.

The dinners began with alternating grandchildren saying some version of "God is good, God is great, thank you for our food. Amen."

Bill always showed pleasure at another tradition that we continued up until the final months of his disease. Our Christmas Eve gala of the year goes back many years, and is captured on a family video of "Christmases Past" that daughter-in-law Donna shot, edited and compiled for us.

Before our sons left the nest, the buffet was for our friends and their friends with a holiday party atmosphere. When our sons married, members of the extended family joined us, and when the grandchildren arrived the party agenda changed into a big family affair.

The food was out early for "grazing" and conversation. Bill's brother Jac and his wife Jan and their two sons, Jackie and Jeremy, traveled from their home in Bethesda, Maryland to join us, and later our niece and great nephew also came from Martha's Vineyard, Massachusetts.

It was our time for exchanging presents, and for the grandchildren to have a preview before they spent Christmas morning in their own homes opening their Santa Clause bounty.

They had seen Santa the night before riding down our street on a fire truck—a Christmas present from our town.

There were piles of discarded wrapping paper amid the greenery of balsam and pine boughs that Bill and I used to adorn the house.

The ceiling high tree blinked its lights as some of the revelers in their Santa hats or reindeer headbands grew weary—and went home.

Among the many memories, two special nights stand out.

The Christmas Eve that Donna and Bill announced their engagement made it an especially exciting evening that took on new meaning. Our family was growing and that was emotionally rewarding for me as an addition to the things that had been missing in my earlier life.

A few years later, their first daughter, Leanna, caused a stir of her own. Bill and I had shopped to find a perfect gift for her, and thought that we had succeeded.

When she opened the big box and got a first glimpse of the rug that featured a friendly dog head, she took one look with a priceless look of awe on her face—and fled. She gradually warmed up to her new pet, as that year's video reports. By the next morning in her home, she is shown opening presents with one hand and patting her new friend with the other.

I was so grateful to have this time of remembering because it was disappearing slowly but surely, and at this point Bill could still appreciate listening even though he could not hang onto anything very long. It is the saddest thing about Alzheimer's because remembering is what gives life a dimension beyond living in the moment.

As the disease progressed beyond the middle, his language skills began to fail and his pronunciation faltered, he searched for words to express his thoughts. His comprehension was diminishing and disorientation was increasing.

He would ask me "What day is it?", "Where are we?", "What time is it?" He could no longer tell time and had lost his ability to read or to write his name. He was unable to recognize our neighbors and that bothered him a lot. It took patience to try to overcome the frustration and I was stressed but I tried to keep it from him. I owed him that for his admirable handling of his disease.

He had forgotten that he had Alzheimer's, but sometimes he would say "I think there is something wrong with me." A comment that sent a chill through me.

Even though it begins with short term memory loss, Alzheimer's goes backward and by now Bill was losing memories of our life together and my sadness intensified. The fabric of our shared life was unraveling as he lost the awareness of the wonders and trials of our married life—and I began to feel alone. I knew I gave him his feeling of security but now I was feeling insecure.

My commitment to making our quality of life the best it could be made it difficult to fill the long days in a meaningful way, but we were always together as his world grew smaller and smaller. I was his link to life.

Now restlessness and pacing made it hard to keep up with him. I was at his side even in our home to protect him from possible harm. He enjoyed tea and always tried to put the tea kettle on the stove. Our stove is electric so I could quickly intervene before disaster ensued. He would try to put things back in their usual places, but it never worked. When I tried to find something it would be in a strange place. Sugar might be in the china cabinet and milk in the cold oven. I wanted to allow him to do as much as he could in my efforts to preserve some of his self esteem.

When I started becoming dysfunctional and accident prone, I realized that I had to take better care of myself if I was going to be here for him. I fell and cut my eyelid enough to require stitches. Then I got full-blown hypochondria, turning every little ache or pain into major diseases like brain tumor, cancer and heart attacks, but my biggest fear was of having a paralyzing stroke. What would we do then?

Financial concerns took hold of me as I wondered if we had enough money for the duration. At first I became a miser but soon reduced it to being frugal. We were never big spenders but we had enjoyed a comfortable life style, and I knew that now there would be big expenses in our future.

I was forced to think of things I had not thought of before that were painful, but necessary. I prepaid his funeral—the most difficult expenditure of my life.

The last few years of his Alzheimer's everything changed drastically for the worst. Bill began pacing and talking constantly—and he was paranoid. His entire focus was on me and he hovered over me, following me from room to room. He ranted day and night and everything he said was distorted. He became untypically complaining and stubborn.

He was completely mixed up. He either wanted to change his clothes five times a day or refused to change them. He was totally uncooperative and sometimes screamed at me. I became so depressed that I thought I would have a nervous breakdown.

Only a small percentage of people with Alzheimer's become violent and Bill never went there. Nice people can usually remain nice with the proper medication.

Bill's doctor prescribed an anti-anxiety drug which calmed him down, but I feared that his personality had changed forever.

When his doctor changed his medication it turned out to be our salvation. He became his self again and I was grateful to have him back. But, he was changing and I could visualize his brain cells dying.

During this "crazy" period, my depression had taken its toll on me but my compassion for him had grown. Trying to adjust to all the drastic changes that were taking place eroded my coping ability and I had to fight depression. I began to feel sorry for myself—and alone. I had lost initiative and energy. I was so tired! One day I lost my cool with him and immediately felt disloyal, but when he meekly asked "Are you mad at me?" my spirit returned.

Our life had become a nightmare—and I couldn't let that happen.

With the help of his new medication and his remarkable spirit, I was able to make new resolves.

Moving back toward the triumph of his basic personality made it possible for us to withstand the continuing deterioration of his mental and physical abilities—and our life continued.

When Bill blankly looked at me and said, "Who are you?" I thought the world had come to an end. I thank God that I heard these saddest of words only a couple of times.

As simplistic as it seems, counting my blessings did help and renewed my dedication to not mourning what we were losing but to celebrate the life we still had.

During these last years, my sanity seemed to be hanging by a thread. Living was almost as hard as it gets, but when a good day came along, I cherished it because I knew there were not many left.

I now had to shower, shave and dress him. He didn't like the shower water hitting him and complained, "It's cold" so it took time and diplomacy to get it done. Even though I had to learn how to shave a man's face, it turned out to be a pleasant experience and a highlight of the day. He would keep smiling at me and I kept telling him that he had to stop so I could do it, and then he would say, "You're beautiful." At these times the Alzheimer's stare disappeared and I saw the familiar face of all our years.

Dressing him was another matter. When I turned around to get another piece of clothing, he would try to remove some other garment. It was a major task trying to put on his socks and shoes because he curled his toes. Distraction was the only thing that helped in these situations.

Comprehension quickly came and went. He moved back and forth from agitation to blank stares when I could see in his eyes that his mind was not working. It was scary and made me feel alone. I missed the old twinkle in his eyes.

The only people he recognized were our immediate family and he couldn't remember much about us except that we were a part of him.

He was usually exhausted before 7 PM but he wouldn't go to bed unless I was there too. I was his security blanket. Walking had become so difficult that one night he couldn't remember or figure out how to move his legs to go up the six steps to the bedroom level. Those few steps must have looked like Mt. Everest to him. It took both of us to get him into bed.

The Alzheimer's years were the final part of our life journey together. Commitment and courage brought us through the worst times, and my perception of the disease made a difference in how we were able to go on.

I was determined to keep him home with me, as I vowed to take care of him for the rest of his life. I could never desert him when he needed me the most.

When he suddenly developed that high fever that took us to the emergency room at 3 AM—a frantic ambulance ride to Mountainside Hospital—it had become obvious from his advanced inabilities that he was in the final stage of Alzheimer's. It was a terrible omen.

Son Bill had been able to spend a great deal of time at our home, helping me to care for his father and saving me from becoming unable to cope with the increased difficulties.

At the hospital, Bill was immediately put on an IV to stabilize him while they made the diagnosis of an infected gall bladder. It was gangrenous and had to be removed.

Bill came through the operation, but the anesthetic probably advanced the Alzheimer's, a theory I had heard from doctors. I remember one saying, "Something usually happens, an accident or another disease surfacing" before someone dies of Alzheimer's, and he hinted that it would be the good news because by that time all quality of life would be gone. I tried to find solace in that prediction.

When Bill was in the hospital there was a slight chance he might go back to where he had been in his disease—but that didn't happen. If the operation had not been necessary he might have lived longer but his quality of life would have hit bottom.

One afternoon when my sadness took over and tears were running down my cheeks, I got on the hospital elevator and recognized one of Bill's resident doctors. When we go off the elevator, he put his arm around my shoulder and offered the kindest words that touched the part of me that was in need. It boosted my failing courage because a crisis situation is a lonely place to be. The four weeks he remained in the hospital, Bill often said "Let's go home." I joined him in wanting one thing—to have him home with me.

The day he came home from the hospital was total chaos. Equipment began arriving, first the hospital bed where he would spend the last four months of his life, and then the walker, lift and wheelchair that he would not be able to use.

Then came all the people, a physical therapist, RN's, aids and social workers from the agencies. They all had questions and forms that put me in a state of confusion.

The first two days home he was disoriented and didn't realize that he was at home so I called our family doctor who prescribed a new medication that briefly brought back some awareness. While it is not possible to change the disease, Alzheimer's can be managed with the right amount of the right medication. Bill was usually on a low enough dosage so that he could be with us as much as his diminished mind permitted.

That winter was an especially snowy one to add to my depression. But every little gesture of caring helped. I particularly remember the night I looked out the window and saw three small figures shoveling the snow in our driveway. They turned out to be the young children of our wonderful next door neighbors. It's impossible to express how much this meant to me.

We always followed Duke basketball, and I had the bedroom television on low the night they won the national championship in 2001. I hoped it might touch a spark, but Bill's love of our alma mater was gone.

Bill died a few days later.

PART V
Aftermath

The loss of Bill is the worst thing that ever happened in my life, at least half of me is gone, and I will never be the same. He will always be a part of me because love never dies, but I am alive—and it is my responsibility to live. There is no option.

His emotional support during our years together made me a better person, and I learned life lessons from him. He instinctively knew what to value in life. He loved people, he loved life and he saw beauty in everything. These are legacies he left me.

The numbness I had for the first couple of years after his death rescued me from devastation. My lack of awareness was as Bill's had been in his illness, and it gave me insight into what it must have been like for him. I just walked through my life, not really being a part of it, or fully aware of what I was doing.

I ate but food had no taste. It was just a necessity so I subsisted on take out. I tried to sleep but I had nightmares and woke up every couple of hours, and was usually up at 4 AM. Our house was cold, empty and quiet, and I kept thinking of things to tell Bill—but I was alone. Aloneness was a paralyzing feeling that I had to fight.

I went to Boston University for my granddaughter's graduation, I went to the Jersey shore with family members, I went to Maryland for a nephew's wedding, I went to a bereavement meeting, and I went to a Broadway show and saw the Manhattan that I had commuted to for over twenty-five years—but had not visited for ten years. These excursions made me feel a little less isolated and made my life bearable, thanks to my attentive family.

Trying to keep my sanity, I forced myself to go to my new write group in Montclair and to my exercise class. I kept the television and radio on during all my waking hours just so I would hear a human voice. The most desolate alone time was when the sun began to set. Ordinary conversation with Bill was a major loss. All during the day, I kept thinking of things to tell him. There were times when I had a feeling of his presence—and then I would realize that I was alone.

I couldn't have the one thing I wanted—Bill.

It was so painful to open his closet and see his clothing still hanging there or to open a kitchen cabinet and see his favorite mugs, especially the "best grandpa" one.

The void was so deep that I didn't see how I would ever be able to function again.

About three years after Bill's death when some of my numbness began to subside, I began my fight with depression. As I began to feel again instead of just being an observer of life, I had to draw on self analysis to believe that I might ever become "normal" again. I couldn't focus. I couldn't think. I couldn't concentrate. Everything was unreal.

It was more painful than before. I was in limbo between denial and reality as I tried to balance emotion and intellect.

When the fog really began to lift and I became able to some degree to interact and relate to other people, I was over-sensitive and fragile.

The first night after Bill's death, I couldn't bear to go into our bedroom, where he had died. It was full of raw emotion even in my unreal state. I decided to temporarily sleep in Phil's old room across the hall, which was as he left it after his marriage many years before. The bookshelves are filled with textbooks and all the literature a future journalist would accumulate—and his old single bed is low on the floor. Sometimes the room echoes the late-night discussions between him and his best friend on politics, ethics and other weighty subjects.

The room became my "dorm room" and still is five years later.

I am now able to go into our old master bedroom without a feeling of horror, but somehow it is not our room anymore. Yet, I can imagine the sanctuary it was for us during all those years.

Gradually I moved some of my clothes into Phil's old chest of drawers and closet. I put my new lavender linens on the single mattress which was badly sagging from wear. It took a couple of years before I had the strength to shop for a new mattress.

The room has become a place to live in my beloved but empty house.

Every day as I pass the photo display from the funeral home that hangs in the hallway on the way to my "dorm room," I pause to enjoy Bill's smile that is also etched in my mind like sunshine, and to appreciate the memories it evokes. The pictures of family events make me smile, and inspire my day with the knowledge that a life full of love is an accomplished life.

When I realized the extent of neglect our home had suffered, there were things to do. After the many expenses of Bill's illness, I had become more frugal and fearful of spending money on our home, and only had essential repairs that had gone undone during those years that my concentration had been on Bill's well being.

When part of the main bathroom ceiling fell through, it became apparent that a new roof was needed for our home. When a letter from the city informed me that I had to have my house painted, I was beginning to feel like a victim, until I discovered the "purplish" paint that looks different hues in different lights to please an artist's eye. My family appreciated it. So would Bill.

Now, I can sit in our home with tranquility and feel the warmth that lives here because our fulfilled lives made it our family history.

As much as I wanted to, I couldn't bring myself to view the Christmas video for a long time, even though the family buffet is still an annual event. It is indescribable to watch Bill in life, which makes the video a treasure for all time.

Rather than think of the Alzheimer's years as a "long death," it was the "in sickness" part of our marriage. If I could have stopped the film in middle disease we could have grown very old together. When I see an old couple hand in hand helping each other, I am touched with envy.

I began to reflect on what had made our marriage work.

Bill and I were different in many ways, but we were alike on the important goals of life, with our number on priority being our family.

Our shared attitude about money was that its only purpose is to provide a comfortable life. We believed that too much excessive wealth is wasted on the wrong things and that ambitions should have a more ethical purpose. Bill never felt a need for luxuries or status symbols. My needs are modest and I am frugal.

Admittedly, if it can classify as a luxury, our first new car, a white Chevy Impala convertible with red interior had seduced us. I think it was just the fun it provided. Our sons have vivid childhood memories of riding down the Garden State Parkway with the top down as we all sang and their grandfather strummed on his ukulele, attracting a lot of attention.

Our shared interest was being with people, and it was a common denominator that helped bond us. Bill's upbeat personality spoke for him and endeared him to the neighborhood, from the pre-teen girls who always brought him valentines to the neighbor he helped gain his citizenship.

We were both sentimentalists who shared our memories and even after his were locked inside him, escaping through his smile, his emotional memory remained.

Bill loved life and was at peace with everything, I think his survival skill in fighting his disease was because of his enviable attitude. His genuine good-will shone through so that people were instinctively drawn to him.

Instead of only thinking of the Alzheimer's years, I am finally able to go back and remember Bill before his disease—the warm person who made everyone feel respected and appreciated.

I can't remember what our arguments were about, but I know that there were no silent treatments that are so often barriers to communication. I was the venter and Bill listened without being judgmental, and when I lost my cool, he was the stabilizer.

When I am troubled, I "talk" to Bill and I can "hear" him "saying," everything will be all right.

Losing a spouse changes everything, and is so debilitating that recovery seems impossible, but I still have life to live. I'm a realist with a dreamer streak who needed the nourishment that Bill gave to me. Emotional wounds, just like physical wounds, need treatment. My life can never be the same but it is up to me to give it purpose.

I stow away my memories, like a squirrel stows away food for the winter, and draw upon them when the going gets tough.

During his disease I was his link to the life we had lived. The consistency of being with me made it real to him because I was indelible in his dysfunctional brain.

His touches with the past, as fleeting as they were, I gave to him like presents—the best I had ever been able to give him. My being with him gave him a life.

Bill knew me better than anyone ever has, and he looked deep inside me to find the things that made him want to spend his life with me.

We had somehow found the person whose presence brought us through whatever life dealt. Call it fate, call it an accident, call it luck, but for us it was a reality. Our marriage was a mutual support system beyond "being there." Giving to each other was the constant element of our relationship that endured.

We were blessed to have all those years to grow closer than ever. I can't make new memories for him, but I have to make new memories for me.

Bill was not "crazy."

Bill was not "a child."

He was always my husband.

and I know
"everything will be all right"

Epilogue

Until the city fulfills its promise to plant another cherry blossom tree, the void remains. But I can envision the beautiful sapling that will share its glorious blossoms with us, as it proudly lives beside the remains of its ancestor to remind the human species that we move into eternity through those who follow us.

About The Author

Glory Read began her writing career as a North Carolina journalist. After having her two sons, she was recruited as a writer for the News Bureau and public relations office at her alma mater, Duke University.

After the family moved to her husband's native New Jersey, she worked in New York as an advertising copywriter, an editor, a newspaper columnist and free lance magazine writer.

For some twenty-five years she was president of Public Relations Counsel, Inc., a Manhattan public relations agency. She was listed in "Who's Who in Public Relations," "Who's Who in the East," and "Foremost Women in Communications."

She created the "Baby Yourself" concept of adult use of baby products. The success of this public relations program was responsible for the development of an adult usage advertising campaign, reported in trade publications as a marketing coup.

She lives in Clifton, N.J. in a purple house near her two sons, Bill an artist and Phil a journalist, and their artistic families.

She is an active member of The Write Group in Montclair, N.J.

Thanks

to the student technicians and medical students at Duke Hospital (where I worked for a year between high school and college) who adopted me as a "sister" and put pressure on me to enroll at Duke.

to the admissions officers at Duke who decided that my heartfelt essay qualified me for admission.

to all the good bosses of my life who believed that women have brains too.

mentors all

and to the admired writers who read my manuscript, encouraged me, and helped to make the telling of my story possible.

and to The Write Group in Montclair, N.J.

and to my son Bill who made this book possible.

Resources

The National Alzheimer's Disease Association is the major source of information and literature. They can give you the name of your local chapter that will acquaint you with all of their many programs, as well as direct you to other services available in your area.

A portion of the profits from this book will be donated to Alzheimer's research.

William M. Read III, protector of water

BY RUSSELL BEN-ALI
STAR-LEDGER STAFF

They were charged with cleaning up the Passaic — no easy task even for a crew of chemists and engineers with a penchant for testing water samples into the night and making after-hour river visits in pursuit of polluters.

But in the years that William Read and his team were responsible for testing the water quality of the river and its watershed, the tests showed that the condition of the Passaic River improved.

"He had a very, very significant position of responsibility — serving water to the equivalent of a million people," said Wendell Inhoffer, a retired general superintendent and chief engineer at the Passaic Valley Water Commission, where Mr. Read worked for 34 years as a chemist, supervisor of research and assistant chief of water quality.

"He was not a 9 to 5 guy — he'd come in early and leave late, always checking and double-checking ev-

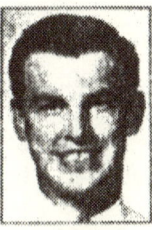

READ

Read's spirit and smile, often maintained despite a harsh illness.

"I want to tell you he was that way until the end," said Glory Read, his wife of 49 years. "Alzheimer's changes some people; not him."

Mr. Read was born in Maywood, said his son, Philip, of Clifton, the West Essex bureau chief for The Star-Ledger.

He graduated from high school in 1942 and attended Duke University in Durham, N.C., but left early to join the Navy, family members said.

Mr. Read took courses at Northwestern University to fulfill the requirements of a Naval officer's training program. He joined the Navy as a commissioned officer, rising to the rank of lieutenant while serving in the Pacific Theater during World War II.

After the war, Mr. Read returned to Duke and earned a bachelor's degree in chemistry, said Glory Read, a writer and journalist who met her husband while pursuing an English degree at Duke.

erything," added Inhoffer. "He was in charge of the complete treatment plant during the days when water quality was a real issue."

William M. Read III, a World War II Naval officer, chemist and water commission executive, died in his Clifton home Monday, after an 11-year bout with Alzheimer's disease. He was 77.

At the Passaic Valley Water Commission in Little Falls, where Mr. Read worked until his 1992 retirement, workers remembered him as an even-handed supervisor.

"He was a very fair man, always very upbeat, very moral, an ethical kind of person," said commission spokeswoman Ethel Senst, who was a laboratory technician while Mr. Read worked as supervisor of research for the river and its source water.

The Passaic Valley Water Commission provides water to Clifton, Passaic and Paterson. Its principal source is the Wanaque Reservoir although some water is obtained from the Passaic River and passes through the commission's treatment plant in Little Falls.

Family members recalled Mr.

The couple married in 1952 and had two sons. They lived in Durham and Hackensack, before settling in Clifton nearly four decades ago.

Mr. Read was a member of the American Chemical Society, the Institute of Chemical Engineers, the Montclair Society of Engineers, the American Water Works Association and the Water Pollution Control Association.

In addition to his wife and son, Mr. Read is survived by another son, William IV of Parsippany; a brother, Jacques of Bethesda, Md., a sister, Diane Haeselbarth of Martha's Vineyard, Mass.; four grandchildren; a niece, two nephews and two great-nephews.

Funeral services will be at 9:15 a.m. today at the Bizub-Quinlan Funeral Home, 1313 Van Houten Ave., Clifton. A 10 a.m. service will follow in St. Peter's Episcopal Church, 380 Clifton Ave., Clifton. Interment will follow in Mount Hebron Cemetery in Upper Montclair.

In lieu of flowers, donations may be made to St. Peter's Haven, Shelter for Homeless Families, 390 Clifton Ave., Clifton, N.J. 07011.

William Marsden Read, III
April 2, 2001

"A beautiful life
that came to an end,
he died as he lived,
everyone's friend.
In our hearts a memory
will always be kept,
of one we loved,
and will never forget."

978-0-595-44006-1
0-595-44006-1